HEALING WITH CASTOR Oil

Unlock and Harness the Power of Nature's Miracle Solution for Holistic Health, Wellness, and Beauty

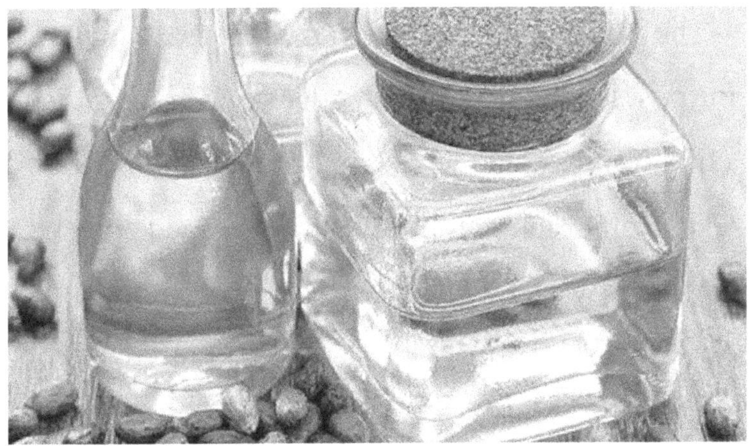

Katherine Peters

Copyright © 2024 by Katherine Peters

The information in this book is for educational purposes only. It is not intended to diagnose, treat, cure, or prevent any disease or medical condition. The author and publisher are not responsible for any adverse effects or consequences resulting from the use of the information contained in this book.

Table of Contents

Part I   **6**

Unlocking the Secrets of Castor Oil   **6**

Chapter 1   7

A Timeless Remedy: The History and Science of Castor Oil   7

Ancient Origins and Traditional Uses   7

Ancient Egypt: A Gift from the Nile   7

Classical Greece: A Panacea for Many Ailments 8

Ancient India: A Holistic Approach to Health   9

Eastern Wisdom: Castor Oil in Traditional Chinese Medicine and Ayurveda   9

Ayurveda: The Science of Life   10

The Science Behind the Magic: Understanding Ricinoleic Acid   12

The Chemistry and Power of Healing   12

The Mechanism of Action   13

How Ricinoleic Acid Works   14

Part II   **16**

Naturally Radiant Skin   **16**

Chapter 2   17

A Skincare Revolution: Castor Oil for Glowing Skin   17

The Secret to Youthful Skin: Hydration and Nourishment   17

Hydration, Hydration, Hydration   17

Nourishing the Skin from Within   18

How to Incorporate Castor Oil into Your Skincare Routine   20

DIY Castor Oil Skincare Recipes   21

Castor oil, with its remarkable hydrating and nourishing properties, is a versatile ingredient that can be incorporated into a variety of DIY skincare recipes. By creating your own skincare products, you can tailor them to your specific needs and avoid harsh chemicals found in many commercial products.   21

Additional Tips for Using Castor Oil in Your Skincare Routine   24

Tailoring Castor Oil for Your Skin Type   25

Oily Skin   25

Dry Skin   26

Sensitive Skin   26

Combination Skin   27

Chapter 3   29

Healing the Skin: Targeting Specific Concerns   29

Clear Skin, Clear Mind: Castor Oil for Acne-Prone Skin   29

How to Use Castor Oil for Acne   30

Important Considerations   31

Additional Tips for Acne-Prone Skin   31

Soothing Sensitive Skin: Castor Oil for Eczema and Psoriasis   32

Castor Oil for Eczema   32

Castor Oil for Psoriasis   33

Turning Back Time: Castor Oil for Youthful Skin   34

How to Use Castor Oil for Anti-Aging   36

Additional Tips for Youthful Skin   36

Part III   **38**

Effortlessly Luscious Locks   **38**

   Chapter 4   39

   Hair, Hair, Don't Care: Castor Oil for Hair Growth and
Health   39

      Scalp Bliss: The Power of Castor Oil Massage   39

         The Role of Castor Oil in Scalp Massage   39

      A Step-by-Step Guide to Nourishing Your Locks
with Castor Oil   41

      Tailoring Castor Oil for Your Unique Hair Type   44

         Straight Hair   44

         Wavy Hair   45

         Curly Hair   45

         Coily Hair   46

   Chapter 5   47

   The Beauty of Natural Hair: Castor Oil for Curls and
Coils   47

      Defining Your Curls: The Power of Castor Oil   47

      Sealing the Deal: Locking in Moisture with Castor
Oil   49

      Deep Conditioning with Castor Oil: A Luxurious
Hair Treatment   52

Part IV   **55**

Total Well-being, Inside and Out   **55**

   Chapter 6   56

   A Healthier You: Castor Oil for Internal Cleansing and
Detoxification   56

      A Gentle Cleanse: Castor Oil for Digestive Health
56

      A Natural Detox: Castor Oil for Liver Health   58

      A Slimmer You: Castor Oil and Weight Loss   61

Chapter 7   64

Pain Relief, Naturally: Castor Oil for Aches and Pains
64

    Soothing Inflammation: The Anti-Inflammatory
    Power of Castor Oil   64

    The Healing Power of Castor Oil Packs   66

Part V   **69**

Your Journey to Holistic Health   **69**

Chapter 8   70

Safety, Precautions, and Common Questions   70

    Understanding the Potential Side Effects of Castor
    Oil   70

        When to Avoid Castor Oil   72

    Debunking Myths: The Truth About Castor Oil   72

Part I

Unlocking the Secrets of Castor Oil

Chapter 1

A Timeless Remedy: The History and Science of Castor Oil

Ancient Origins and Traditional Uses

Castor oil, derived from the seeds of the castor plant, *Ricinus communis* boasts a rich and storied history, dating back thousands of years. Its unique properties and versatile applications have made it a prized commodity in various ancient civilizations.

Ancient Egypt: A Gift from the Nile

In the heart of ancient Egypt, along the fertile banks of the Nile River, castor oil was revered as a potent remedy. Egyptian physicians and healers recognized its therapeutic value and incorporated it into their medicinal practices.

- **Beauty Elixir**: Egyptian women prized castor oil for its ability to enhance beauty. It was used to nourish the skin, promote hair growth, and maintain a youthful appearance.

- **Healing Ointment**: Castor oil was a key ingredient in ointments used to treat wounds, burns, and skin infections. Its antimicrobial properties helped to prevent infection and promote healing.
- **Sacred Rituals**: Castor oil also played a role in ancient Egyptian religious rituals. It was used in anointing ceremonies and as an offering to the gods.

Classical Greece: A Panacea for Many Ailments

The ancient Greeks, renowned for their contributions to medicine and philosophy, also recognized the therapeutic potential of castor oil.

- **A Remedy for Digestive Disorders**: Greek physicians prescribed castor oil as a laxative to alleviate constipation and other digestive issues.
- **Topical Applications**: Castor oil was used topically to treat skin conditions, such as eczema and psoriasis.
- **Wound Care**: It was also applied to wounds to promote healing and prevent infection.

Ancient India: A Holistic Approach to Health

In the ancient Indian subcontinent, castor oil was an integral part of the Ayurvedic system of medicine.

- **Ayurvedic Remedies**: Ayurvedic practitioners used castor oil to treat a wide range of ailments, including headaches, joint pain, and respiratory infections.
- **Hair Care**: Castor oil was a popular hair treatment, used to strengthen hair follicles, prevent hair loss, and promote hair growth.
- **Skin Care**: It was also used to nourish the skin, reduce wrinkles, and improve complexion.

The ancient Egyptians, Greeks, and Indians, among other civilizations, recognized the remarkable properties of castor oil. Their knowledge and wisdom, passed down through generations, have contributed to the enduring legacy of this versatile natural remedy.

Eastern Wisdom: Castor Oil in Traditional Chinese Medicine and Ayurveda

Castor oil, with its rich history and diverse applications, has also been a cornerstone of traditional Chinese medicine (TCM) and Ayurveda. These ancient systems of medicine recognized the plant's therapeutic potential and incorporated it into various remedies to address a wide range of health concerns.

In traditional Chinese medicine, castor oil, known as "Ba Dou You," is considered a potent remedy with a wide range of applications. It is believed to have a warming nature and can be used to treat a variety of ailments, including:

- **Digestive Disorders**: Castor oil is used to alleviate constipation and other digestive issues. It is believed to stimulate the intestines and promote regular bowel movements.
- **Pain Relief**: In TCM, castor oil is applied topically to relieve pain associated with arthritis, muscle aches, and joint pain. It is also used to reduce inflammation and swelling.
- **Skin Conditions**: Castor oil is used to treat various skin conditions, such as eczema, psoriasis, and acne. It is believed to soothe the skin, reduce inflammation, and promote healing.
- **Respiratory Disorders**: Castor oil is used to treat respiratory conditions, such as coughs, colds, and bronchitis. It is believed to help clear the lungs and sinuses.

Ayurveda: The Science of Life

In Ayurveda, castor oil, known as "Eranda Taila," is considered a powerful medicinal herb. It is used to treat a wide range of health conditions, including:

- **Digestive Disorders**: Ayurvedic practitioners use castor oil to treat constipation, indigestion, and other digestive issues. It is believed to stimulate the digestive fire and improve digestion.
- **Skin Disorders**: Castor oil is used to treat various skin conditions, such as acne, eczema, and psoriasis. It is believed to soothe the skin, reduce inflammation, and promote healing.
- **Hair Care**: Castor oil is widely used in Ayurvedic hair care. It is believed to nourish the hair follicles, prevent hair loss, and promote hair growth.
- **Pain Relief**: Castor oil is used to relieve pain associated with arthritis, muscle aches, and joint pain. It is also used to reduce inflammation and swelling.
- **Detoxification**: Ayurvedic practitioners use castor oil for detoxification purposes. It is believed to help remove toxins from the body and promote overall health.

Both traditional Chinese medicine and Ayurveda recognize the therapeutic potential of castor oil. Its ability to address a wide range of health concerns, from digestive issues to skin problems, has made it a valuable remedy for centuries. As we continue to explore the science behind castor oil, we can appreciate the wisdom of these ancient systems of medicine and their enduring legacy.

The Science Behind the Magic: Understanding Ricinoleic Acid

At the heart of castor oil's therapeutic properties lies a unique fatty acid known as ricinoleic acid. This compound, which makes up approximately 90% of the fatty acids in castor oil, is responsible for many of its beneficial effects.

The Chemistry and Power of Healing

Ricinoleic acid is an 18-carbon unsaturated fatty acid with a hydroxyl group attached to the 12th carbon atom. This unique chemical structure gives ricinoleic acid several distinctive properties, including:

- **Hydrating Properties**: Ricinoleic acid is highly moisturizing, making it an excellent ingredient for skin and hair care products. It helps to retain moisture, preventing dryness and promoting a healthy, youthful appearance.
- **Anti-inflammatory Effects**: Ricinoleic acid has potent anti-inflammatory properties. It helps to reduce inflammation in the body, which can alleviate pain and discomfort associated with conditions such as arthritis, muscle aches, and skin inflammation.

- **Antimicrobial Activity**: Ricinoleic acid exhibits antimicrobial properties, which means it can help to kill bacteria, fungi, and other harmful microorganisms. This makes it effective in treating skin infections and promoting wound healing.
- **Laxative Effect**: Ricinoleic acid stimulates the muscles in the intestines, promoting bowel movements and relieving constipation. However, it is important to use castor oil as a laxative under the guidance of a healthcare professional.
- **Pain Relief**: Ricinoleic acid can help to relieve pain by blocking pain signals and reducing inflammation. It is often used to alleviate pain associated with muscle aches, joint pain, and headaches.

The Mechanism of Action

The exact mechanism of action of ricinoleic acid is not fully understood, but researchers believe that it works through a variety of pathways. Some of the proposed mechanisms include:

- **Direct Inhibition of Inflammatory Pathways**: Ricinoleic acid may directly inhibit the production of inflammatory substances, such as prostaglandins and cytokines.
- **Activation of Cellular Repair Mechanisms**: Ricinoleic acid may stimulate the body's natural

healing processes, promoting the growth of new cells and tissues.

- **Modulation of Immune Response**: Ricinoleic acid may help to regulate the immune system, reducing inflammation and promoting healing.

How Ricinoleic Acid Works

Ricinoleic acid works in several ways to promote health and well-being:

- **Topical Application**: When applied topically, ricinoleic acid can penetrate the skin and exert its therapeutic effects. It can reduce inflammation, soothe irritation, and promote healing.
- **Oral Consumption**: When taken orally, ricinoleic acid can stimulate the intestines and promote bowel movements. It can also help to reduce inflammation in the digestive tract.
- **Systemic Effects**: Ricinoleic acid can be absorbed into the bloodstream and exert systemic effects. It can help to reduce inflammation throughout the body and promote overall health.

By understanding the role of ricinoleic acid, we can appreciate the full potential of castor oil. Its unique chemical structure and diverse properties make it a valuable ingredient in a wide range of natural remedies. As research continues to explore the full potential of ricinoleic acid, it is likely that we will discover even more ways to harness its power for optimal health and well-being.

Part II

Naturally Radiant Skin

Chapter 2

A Skincare Revolution: Castor Oil for Glowing Skin

The Secret to Youthful Skin: Hydration and Nourishment

Castor oil has long been hailed as a natural beauty elixir, capable of transforming skin from dull and lackluster to radiant and glowing. Its unique properties, particularly its ability to hydrate and nourish the skin, have made it a popular ingredient in skincare routines.

Hydration, Hydration, Hydration

Hydration is essential for maintaining healthy, youthful-looking skin. When the skin is dehydrated, it can become dry, flaky, and prone to premature aging. Ricinoleic acid, a fatty acid found abundantly in castor oil, plays a crucial role in maintaining skin hydration. It acts as a humectant, attracting and retaining moisture from the atmosphere. This helps to prevent moisture loss, keeping the skin soft, supple, and plump. Additionally, ricinoleic acid forms a protective barrier on the skin's surface, shielding it from environmental stressors like pollution, wind, and cold weather. This is particularly beneficial for individuals with dry or dehydrated skin, as it helps to restore the skin's natural moisture balance.

Nourishing the Skin from Within

Beyond hydration, castor oil offers a plethora of nourishing benefits for the skin. Castor oil is rich in essential fatty acids, including ricinoleic acid, which plays a crucial role in skin health. These fatty acids nourish the skin cells, promoting cell turnover and regeneration. They also help to strengthen the skin's barrier function, protecting it from environmental damage and pollutants. Here's how it works:

- **Antioxidant Protection**: Castor oil contains antioxidants that combat free radicals, which are harmful molecules that can damage the skin and accelerate aging. By neutralizing these free radicals, castor oil helps to prevent premature aging, fine lines, and wrinkles.
- **Anti-inflammatory Properties**: Ricinoleic acid possesses anti-inflammatory properties that can soothe irritated skin and reduce redness. It can be particularly beneficial for individuals with sensitive skin or inflammatory skin conditions like eczema and psoriasis.

- **Enhanced Skin Cell Turnover**: Castor oil can help to accelerate the skin's natural cell turnover process. This can lead to a more youthful appearance, as it helps to remove dead skin cells and reveal a fresh, radiant complexion.
- **Improved Skin Texture**: Regular use of castor oil can help to improve the overall texture of the skin. It can smooth out rough patches, minimize the appearance of pores, and leave the skin feeling soft and silky.

By hydrating and nourishing the skin, castor oil can help to improve a variety of skin concerns, including:

- **Dry Skin**: Castor oil can help to alleviate dryness and flakiness, leaving the skin soft, smooth, and supple.
- **Dull Skin**: Castor oil can help to brighten the complexion, giving the skin a radiant glow.
- **Aging Skin**: Castor oil can help to reduce the appearance of fine lines, wrinkles, and age spots.
- **Sensitive Skin**: Castor oil is gentle and non-irritating, making it suitable for sensitive skin.

How to Incorporate Castor Oil into Your Skincare Routine

To reap the benefits of castor oil, you can incorporate castor oil into your skincare routine, you can use it directly on your skin or add it to your favorite skincare products. You can also create your own DIY skincare products using castor oil as a key ingredient

- **Moisturizer**: Apply a few drops of castor oil directly to your face and neck after cleansing. It can be used alone or mixed with other oils or moisturizers.
- **Hair Oil**: Apply castor oil to your scalp and hair, leave it on for a few hours or overnight, and then shampoo it off. This can help to nourish your hair, promote hair growth, and reduce hair breakage.
- **Face Mask**: Mix castor oil with other natural ingredients like honey to create a nourishing face mask.
- **Facial Massage**: Warm a few drops of castor oil and gently massage it into your face in circular motions. This can help to improve blood circulation, reduce puffiness, and promote relaxation.
- **Body Oil**: Use castor oil as a body moisturizer to soften and smooth your skin.

- **Lip Balm**: Mix castor oil with beeswax and essential oils to create a natural, moisturizing lip balm.

By understanding the mechanisms behind castor oil's hydrating and nourishing properties, you can harness its power and effectively incorporate it into your skincare routine to achieve a radiant and glowing complexion.

DIY Castor Oil Skincare Recipes

Castor oil, with its remarkable hydrating and nourishing properties, is a versatile ingredient that can be incorporated into a variety of DIY skincare recipes. By creating your own skincare products, you can tailor them to your specific needs and avoid harsh chemicals found in many commercial products.

Here are a few DIY skincare recipes that harness the power of castor oil:

1. Hydrating Castor Oil Facial Cleanser

- **Ingredients**:
    1. 1/4 cup mild, gentle cleanser (e.g., castile soap, baby shampoo)
    2. 1 tablespoon castor oil

3. 1 teaspoon honey
4. 1 teaspoon vitamin E oil

- **Instructions**:
    1. Combine all ingredients in a small bowl and mix well until a smooth, creamy consistency is achieved.
    2. Wet your face with warm water and gently massage the cleanser onto your skin in circular motions.
    3. Rinse thoroughly with warm water and pat your face dry with a clean towel.

2. Nourishing Castor Oil Moisturizer

- **Ingredients**:
    1. 1/4 cup shea butter
    2. 2 tablespoons coconut oil
    3. 1 tablespoon castor oil
    4. 1 teaspoon jojoba oil
    5. A few drops of your favorite essential oil (optional)
- **Instructions**:
    1. Melt the shea butter and coconut oil together in a double boiler or microwave.
    2. Remove from heat and add the castor oil and jojoba oil.
    3. Stir well until all ingredients are combined.
    4. Add a few drops of your favorite essential oil for fragrance.

5. Transfer the mixture to a clean jar and allow it to cool and solidify.

3. Anti-Aging Castor Oil Face Mask

- **Ingredients**:
    1. 1 tablespoon bentonite clay
    2. 1 tablespoon apple cider vinegar
    3. 1 teaspoon honey
    4. 1 teaspoon castor oil
- **Instructions**:
    1. In a small bowl, combine the bentonite clay, apple cider vinegar, and honey.
    2. Slowly add the castor oil, stirring continuously until a smooth paste forms.
    3. Apply the mask to your clean, dry face, avoiding the eye and lip area.
    4. Leave the mask on for 10-15 minutes, or until it dries completely.
    5. Rinse off with warm water and pat your face dry.

4. Castor Oil Hair Mask

- **Ingredients**:
    1. 2 tablespoons castor oil
    2. 1 tablespoon coconut oil
    3. 1 tablespoon olive oil

- **Instructions**:
    1. Warm the oils together in a microwave or double boiler.
    2. Apply the warm oil mixture to your scalp and hair, massaging gently.
    3. Cover your hair with a shower cap and leave the mask on for at least 30 minutes, or overnight for deeper conditioning.
    4. Shampoo and condition your hair as usual.

Additional Tips for Using Castor Oil in Your Skincare Routine

- **Patch Test**: Before using any new skincare product, including those made with castor oil, it's important to perform a patch test to check for any allergic reactions.
- **Consistency is Key**: To see the best results, incorporate castor oil into your skincare routine consistently.
- **Less is More**: A little castor oil goes a long way. Start with a small amount and adjust as needed.
- **Customize Your Recipes**: Feel free to experiment with different ingredients and ratios to create personalized skincare products that suit your specific needs and preferences.

By incorporating these DIY skincare recipes into your beauty regimen, you can harness the power of castor oil to achieve a radiant, youthful complexion. Remember, consistency is key, so stick to your routine and enjoy the benefits of this natural wonder.

Tailoring Castor Oil for Your Skin Type

Castor oil, with its unique blend of fatty acids and antioxidants, offers a wide range of benefits for various skin types. While it may seem like a one-size-fits-all solution, understanding your specific skin type and tailoring your skincare routine accordingly is crucial. Let's explore how castor oil can be beneficial for different skin types:

Oily Skin

Oily skin is prone to breakouts, acne, and a shiny appearance. While it may seem counterintuitive to add oil to oily skin, castor oil can actually help balance sebum production. Here's how:

- **Regulates Sebum Production**: Castor oil helps to regulate the sebaceous glands, which produce sebum, the natural oil that keeps your skin moisturized. By balancing sebum production, castor oil can help to reduce the appearance of oily skin and prevent breakouts.
- **Antimicrobial Properties**: Castor oil has antimicrobial properties that can help to fight

bacteria that cause acne. By applying a small amount of castor oil directly to blemishes, you can help to reduce inflammation and promote healing.

- **Deep Cleansing:** When used as a cleanser, castor oil can effectively remove dirt, makeup, and excess oil without stripping the skin of its natural moisture.

Dry Skin

Dry skin often feels tight, flaky, and itchy. Castor oil's hydrating and nourishing properties make it an excellent choice for those with dry skin.

- **Deep Hydration**: Castor oil penetrates deep into the skin, providing intense hydration. It helps to lock in moisture, preventing dryness and flakiness.
- **Soothes Dry, Irritated Skin**: Castor oil's anti-inflammatory properties can help to soothe dry, irritated skin and reduce redness.
- **Softens and Smooths**: Regular use of castor oil can help to soften and smooth rough, dry patches of skin.

Sensitive Skin

Sensitive skin is prone to redness, irritation, and allergic reactions. Castor oil, when used in moderation, can be gentle on sensitive skin.

- **Soothing and Calming**: Castor oil's anti-inflammatory properties can help to soothe sensitive skin and reduce redness.
- **Hydration Without Irritation**: Castor oil provides gentle hydration without irritating sensitive skin.
- **Natural Barrier Protection**: Castor oil can help to strengthen the skin's natural barrier, protecting it from environmental stressors.

Combination Skin

Combination skin has both oily and dry areas. Castor oil can be beneficial for balancing the skin and addressing both concerns.

- **Hydrates Dry Patches**: Apply castor oil to dry areas of the skin, such as the cheeks, to provide deep hydration.
- **Balances Oily Areas:** Use a small amount of castor oil on oily areas, such as the T-zone, to help regulate sebum production.

Remember, when using castor oil on your face, it's important to start with a small amount and gradually increase as needed. Patch testing is also recommended to ensure you don't have any adverse reactions. If you have any concerns or specific skin conditions, consult with a dermatologist before using castor oil.

Chapter 3

Healing the Skin: Targeting Specific Concerns

Clear Skin, Clear Mind: Castor Oil for Acne-Prone Skin

Acne, a common skin condition characterized by pimples, blackheads, and whiteheads, can significantly impact self-esteem and quality of life. While there are numerous over-the-counter and prescription treatments available, many people are turning to natural remedies like castor oil to address their acne concerns.

Understanding the Science Behind the Benefits

Castor oil's efficacy in treating acne can be attributed to its unique properties:

- **Anti-inflammatory Properties**: Ricinoleic acid, the primary fatty acid in castor oil, possesses potent anti-inflammatory properties. When applied topically, it can help reduce inflammation, redness, and swelling associated with acne.

- **Antimicrobial Activity**: Castor oil exhibits antimicrobial properties, which means it can help to kill bacteria that contribute to acne breakouts. By targeting these bacteria, castor oil can help to prevent future breakouts.
- **Sebum Regulation**: Castor oil can help to regulate sebum production, the oily substance produced by the skin's sebaceous glands. Excess sebum can clog pores and lead to acne. By balancing sebum production, castor oil can help to prevent future breakouts.

How to Use Castor Oil for Acne

There are several ways to incorporate castor oil into your skincare routine to target acne:

- **Spot Treatment**: Apply a small amount of castor oil directly to individual pimples using a cotton swab. Leave it on overnight and rinse off in the morning.
- **Facial Mask**: Mix castor oil with other natural ingredients like bentonite clay or honey to create a soothing face mask. Apply the mask to your face, leave it on for 10-15 minutes, and then rinse off with warm water.
- **Cleanser**: Add a few drops of castor oil to your favorite facial cleanser to create a gentle, cleansing formula that can help to remove excess oil and dirt without stripping the skin of its natural moisture.

Important Considerations

While castor oil can be effective in treating acne, it's important to use it correctly and be patient. Here are a few tips:

- **Patch Test**: Before applying castor oil to your face, perform a patch test on a small area of skin to check for any allergic reactions.
- **Start Slow**: Begin by using a small amount of castor oil and gradually increase the amount as needed.
- **Consistent Use**: For optimal results, use castor oil consistently as part of your skincare routine.
- **Consult a Dermatologist**: If you have severe acne or other skin conditions, it's important to consult with a dermatologist for proper diagnosis and treatment.

Additional Tips for Acne-Prone Skin

In addition to using castor oil, here are some additional tips for managing acne-prone skin:

- **Gentle Cleansing:** Wash your face twice a day with a gentle, fragrance-free cleanser.
- **Avoid Over-Washing:** Over-washing your face can strip the skin of its natural oils and lead to increased oil production.

- **Moisturize:** Keep your skin hydrated by using a lightweight, non-comedogenic moisturizer.
- **Protect Your Skin:** Wear sunscreen with an SPF of 30 or higher to protect your skin from the sun's harmful rays.

By incorporating castor oil into your skincare routine, and following these tips, you can help to reduce inflammation, prevent breakouts, and achieve clearer, healthier skin.

Soothing Sensitive Skin: Castor Oil for Eczema and Psoriasis

Eczema and psoriasis are chronic skin conditions that can cause significant discomfort and distress. Characterized by itchy, red, and inflamed skin, these conditions can be challenging to manage. Fortunately, natural remedies like castor oil can offer relief and help to soothe irritated skin.

Castor Oil for Eczema

Eczema, also known as atopic dermatitis, is a common skin condition that causes dry, itchy, and inflamed skin. Castor oil can be a valuable tool in managing eczema symptoms:

- **Hydration**: Castor oil is a potent humectant, meaning it attracts and retains moisture. By deeply hydrating the skin, castor oil can help to alleviate dryness and flakiness, two common symptoms of eczema.

- **Anti-inflammatory Properties**: Castor oil possesses anti-inflammatory properties that can help to reduce inflammation and redness associated with eczema. This can help to soothe irritated skin and alleviate itching.
- **Barrier Repair**: Castor oil can help to strengthen the skin's natural barrier, which helps to prevent moisture loss and protect the skin from irritants.

How to Use Castor Oil for Eczema:

- **Direct Application**: Apply a small amount of castor oil directly to the affected areas of skin. Massage gently to promote absorption.
- **Castor Oil Packs**: Apply a warm castor oil pack to the affected areas. This can help to reduce inflammation and promote healing.
- **Bath Additives**: Add a few drops of castor oil to your bathwater to soothe and hydrate your skin.

Castor Oil for Psoriasis

Psoriasis is a chronic autoimmune disease that causes skin cells to grow too quickly, resulting in thick, scaly patches. Castor oil can help to alleviate symptoms of psoriasis:

- **Anti-inflammatory Effects**: Castor oil's anti-inflammatory properties can help to reduce inflammation and redness associated with psoriasis.

- **Moisturizing Benefits**: Castor oil can help to hydrate the skin and prevent dryness, which can exacerbate psoriasis symptoms.
- **Soothing Itchy Skin**: Castor oil can help to soothe itchy skin, a common symptom of psoriasis.

How to Use Castor Oil for Psoriasis:

- **Topical Application**: Apply a small amount of castor oil directly to the affected areas of skin.
- **Castor Oil Packs**: Use a warm castor oil pack on the affected areas to reduce inflammation and promote healing.
- **Bath Additives**: Add a few drops of castor oil to your bathwater to soothe and hydrate your skin.

While castor oil can be a helpful addition to your skincare routine for eczema and psoriasis, it's important to consult with a healthcare professional for a proper diagnosis and treatment plan. Castor oil may not be suitable for everyone, and it's essential to use it under the guidance of a qualified healthcare provider.

Turning Back Time: Castor Oil for Youthful Skin

As we age, our skin undergoes natural changes, leading to the formation of wrinkles and fine lines. While aging is inevitable, there are ways to slow down the process and maintain a youthful appearance. Castor oil, with its unique properties, can be a valuable tool in your anti-aging skincare routine.

Castor oil's anti-aging benefits can be attributed to its rich composition of fatty acids, antioxidants, and vitamins. Here's how it works:

- **Hydration**: Castor oil is a potent humectant, meaning it attracts and retains moisture. By keeping the skin hydrated, it can help to plump up the skin, reducing the appearance of fine lines and wrinkles.
- **Antioxidant Protection**: Castor oil contains antioxidants that help to neutralize free radicals, which are harmful molecules that can damage the skin and accelerate aging. By combating free radicals, castor oil can help to prevent premature aging.
- **Stimulates Collagen Production**: Collagen is a protein that gives the skin its structure and elasticity. As we age, collagen production declines, leading to sagging skin and wrinkles. Castor oil can help to stimulate collagen production, promoting firmer, more youthful-looking skin.
- **Improved Skin Texture**: Regular use of castor oil can help to improve the overall texture of the skin. It can smooth out rough patches, minimize the appearance of pores, and leave the skin feeling soft and supple.

How to Use Castor Oil for Anti-Aging

To harness the anti-aging benefits of castor oil, you can incorporate it into your skincare routine in the following ways:

- **Nighttime Moisturizer**: Apply a few drops of castor oil to your face and neck before bed. It will penetrate deep into the skin, providing intense hydration and nourishment.
- **Facial Massage**: Warm a few drops of castor oil and gently massage it into your face in circular motions. This can help to improve blood circulation, reduce puffiness, and promote relaxation.
- **Face Mask**: Mix castor oil with other natural ingredients like honey, yogurt, or avocado to create a nourishing face mask. Apply the mask to your face, leave it on for 10-15 minutes, and then rinse off with warm water.

Additional Tips for Youthful Skin

In addition to using castor oil, here are some other tips for maintaining youthful skin:

- **Protect Your Skin from the Sun**: Wear sunscreen with an SPF of 30 or higher every day, even on cloudy days.

- **Eat a Healthy Diet**: A diet rich in fruits, vegetables, and whole grains can help to nourish your skin from within.
- **Stay Hydrated**: Drink plenty of water to keep your skin hydrated.
- **Get Enough Sleep**: Aim for 7-8 hours of sleep each night to allow your skin to repair itself.
- **Manage Stress**: Stress can negatively impact your skin. Practice relaxation techniques like yoga, meditation, or deep breathing to reduce stress.

Part III

Effortlessly Luscious Locks

Chapter 4

Hair, Hair, Don't Care: Castor Oil for Hair Growth and Health

Scalp Bliss: The Power of Castor Oil Massage

A healthy scalp is the foundation of healthy hair. When your scalp is nourished and well-circulated, it can promote hair growth, reduce hair loss, and improve overall hair health. One effective way to achieve this is through regular scalp massages with castor oil.

Scalp massage offers a myriad of benefits for your hair and scalp health. When you massage your scalp, you stimulate the blood flow to the hair follicles. Increased blood flow delivers essential nutrients and oxygen to the hair follicles, promoting hair growth and preventing hair loss.

The Role of Castor Oil in Scalp Massage

Castor oil, with its rich fatty acid content, can enhance the benefits of scalp massage. When combined with a gentle massage, castor oil can:

- **Nourish the Hair Follicles**: Castor oil penetrates deep into the hair follicles, providing essential nutrients like omega-6 fatty acids. These nutrients nourish the hair follicles, promoting hair growth and preventing hair loss.
- **Improve Blood Circulation**: The massaging action, combined with the lubricating properties of castor oil, helps to stimulate blood circulation to the scalp. This increased blood flow delivers vital nutrients and oxygen to the hair follicles, promoting hair growth and strengthening the hair roots.
- **Condition the Hair**: Castor oil coats the hair shaft, providing deep conditioning and hydration. This helps to prevent hair breakage, split ends, and frizz.
- **Soothe the Scalp**: Castor oil has anti-inflammatory properties that can help to soothe an irritated scalp. It can alleviate itching, dryness, and other scalp issues.

How to Perform a Castor Oil Scalp Massage

1. **Warm the Oil**: Gently warm the castor oil to enhance its penetration.
2. **Apply the Oil**: Massage the warm castor oil into your scalp using your fingertips.
3. **Massage Techniques**: Use circular motions, gentle kneading, and pulling motions to stimulate the scalp.
4. **Leave-In Time**: Leave the oil on your scalp for at least 30 minutes, or ideally, overnight.

5. **Rinse Thoroughly**: Shampoo your hair thoroughly to remove the oil.

Additional Tips for Healthy Hair

- **Regular Scalp Massages**: Aim to perform a scalp massage at least once a week.
- **Healthy Diet**: Consume a balanced diet rich in vitamins, minerals, and protein.
- **Gentle Hair Care**: Avoid harsh chemicals and excessive heat styling.
- **Hydration**: Drink plenty of water to keep your hair and scalp hydrated.
- **Stress Management**: Manage stress through relaxation techniques like yoga, meditation, or deep breathing.

By incorporating regular scalp massages with castor oil into your hair care routine, you can nourish your hair follicles, promote hair growth, and achieve healthier, stronger, and more beautiful hair.

A Step-by-Step Guide to Nourishing Your Locks with Castor Oil

Castor oil has long been hailed as a miracle ingredient for hair growth and health. Its rich fatty acid content, particularly ricinoleic acid, deeply nourishes the hair follicles and promotes hair growth. Here's a step-by-step guide on how to incorporate castor oil into your hair care routine:

Step 1: Warm the Oil

- **Gentle Heating**: Warm the castor oil slightly, either by placing the bottle in a bowl of hot water or using a hair dryer on low heat.
- **Optimal Temperature**: Ensure the oil is warm, not hot, to avoid damaging your hair and scalp.

Step 2: Apply to Scalp and Hair

- **Section Your Hair**: Divide your hair into sections to ensure even distribution of the oil.
- **Scalp Massage**: Apply the warm castor oil directly to your scalp and massage it in using your fingertips. This stimulates blood circulation, promoting hair growth and nutrient absorption.
- **Hair Length**: Work the remaining oil through the length of your hair, focusing on the ends to prevent split ends and dryness.

Step 3: Leave-In Treatment

- **Overnight Treatment**: For maximum benefits, leave the oil on your hair overnight. Cover your hair with a shower cap to prevent staining your pillowcase.

- **Shorter Treatment**: If you prefer a shorter treatment, leave the oil on your hair for at least 30 minutes.

Step 4: Wash Your Hair

- **Gentle Cleansing**: Use a gentle, sulfate-free shampoo to wash your hair thoroughly.
- **Thorough Rinse**: Ensure that all the oil is rinsed out to avoid a greasy residue.
- **Conditioning**: Follow up with a conditioner to hydrate and detangle your hair.

Frequency of Application

The frequency of castor oil treatments can vary depending on your hair type and specific needs. However, a general guideline is:

- **For Dry and Damaged Hair:** Apply castor oil once or twice a week.
- **For Normal Hair:** Apply castor oil once every two weeks.
- **For Oily Hair:** Use castor oil sparingly, perhaps once a month, focusing on the scalp.
- **Customize Your Routine**: Adjust the frequency based on your hair's specific needs and how your hair responds to the treatment.

Additional Tips for Maximizing Results

- **Combine with Other Oils**: You can mix castor oil with other hair-friendly oils like coconut oil, olive oil, or argan oil to enhance its benefits.
- **Hot Oil Treatment**: For a deeper conditioning treatment, heat the oil and apply it to your hair and scalp. Cover your hair with a shower cap and leave it on for 30 minutes to an hour.
- **Healthy Diet**: A balanced diet rich in vitamins, minerals, and protein is essential for healthy hair growth.
- **Gentle Hair Care**: Avoid harsh chemicals, excessive heat styling, and tight hairstyles.

Tailoring Castor Oil for Your Unique Hair Type

Castor oil is a versatile hair care ingredient that can benefit a wide range of hair types, from straight to coily. While it's a fantastic choice for most hair types, it's essential to understand how to tailor its use to your specific hair needs. By understanding the specific needs of your hair type, you can harness the power of castor oil to achieve optimal results.

Straight Hair

Straight hair can sometimes lack volume and shine. Castor oil can help to address these concerns:

- **Adds Volume**: Castor oil can help to thicken the hair shaft, giving your hair a fuller, more voluminous appearance.
- **Prevents Hair Loss**: Regular use of castor oil can strengthen the hair roots and prevent hair loss, ensuring a healthy scalp and luscious locks.
- **Adds Shine**: The moisturizing properties of castor oil can help to add shine and luster to straight hair.

Wavy Hair

Wavy hair can be prone to frizz and dryness. Castor oil can help to tame frizz and enhance your natural waves:

- **Tames Frizz**: Castor oil's moisturizing properties can help to smooth the hair cuticle, reducing frizz and flyaways.
- **Defines Curls**: By adding definition to your waves, castor oil can help to create a more polished and defined look.
- **Prevents Breakage**: Regular use of castor oil can help to strengthen the hair shaft, reducing breakage and split ends.

Curly Hair

Curly hair is often delicate and prone to dryness and damage. Castor oil can help to nourish and hydrate curly hair:

- **Deep Conditioning**: Castor oil can deeply condition curly hair, providing essential moisture and preventing dryness.
- **Defines Curls**: By defining the curls and reducing frizz, castor oil can help to enhance your natural curl pattern.
- **Strengthens Hair**: Castor oil can strengthen the hair shaft, reducing breakage and promoting hair growth.

Coily Hair

Coily hair is often the most fragile hair type, requiring extra care and attention. Castor oil can help to nourish and protect coily hair:

- **Moisture Retention**: Castor oil can help to seal in moisture, preventing dryness and breakage.
- **Softens and Detangles**: It can soften the hair, making it easier to detangle and style.
- **Promotes Hair Growth**: Regular use of castor oil can help to stimulate hair growth and promote a healthy scalp.

Remember, when using castor oil, it's important to start with a small amount and gradually increase as needed. You may also want to experiment with different application methods and leave-in times to find what works best for your hair type.

Chapter 5

The Beauty of Natural Hair: Castor Oil for Curls and Coils

Defining Your Curls: The Power of Castor Oil

Curly and coily hair types often require special care to maintain their natural beauty. Castor oil, with its unique properties, can be a game-changer for those with curly and coily hair. It helps to define curls, reduce frizz, and promote healthy hair growth.

Understanding the Benefits of Castor Oil for Curly Hair

- **Deep Conditioning**: Castor oil penetrates the hair shaft, providing deep conditioning and hydration.

This helps to prevent dryness, breakage, and split ends, common issues for curly hair.

- **Defining Curls**: The rich, emollient nature of castor oil helps to define and enhance natural curl patterns. It coats each strand, reducing frizz and promoting a more defined curl.
- **Strengthening Hair**: Castor oil nourishes the hair follicles, strengthening the hair shaft from the root to the tip. This helps to prevent breakage and promotes hair growth.
- **Scalp Health**: Regular scalp massages with castor oil can stimulate blood circulation, promoting a healthy scalp and encouraging hair growth.

How to Use Castor Oil to Define Curls and Reduce Frizz

1. **Pre-Poo Treatment**: Apply a generous amount of castor oil to dry hair, focusing on the ends. Cover your hair with a shower cap and leave it on for several hours or overnight. This pre-poo treatment helps to soften the hair and prepare it for washing.
2. **Deep Conditioning Treatment**: Mix castor oil with other hair oils, such as coconut oil or olive oil, to create a deep conditioning treatment. Apply the mixture to your hair, focusing on the ends. Cover your hair with a shower cap and leave it on for 30 minutes to an hour.
3. **Leave-In Conditioner**: Add a few drops of castor oil to your favorite leave-in conditioner. Apply it to

damp hair, focusing on the ends to seal in moisture and prevent frizz.

4. **Sealant**: After applying your favorite styling products, seal in moisture by applying a small amount of castor oil to the ends of your hair. This will help to prevent dryness and breakage.

Additional Tips for Curly and Coily Hair

- **Low-Manipulation Styles**: Opt for protective hairstyles that minimize manipulation and reduce breakage.
- **Regular Trims**: Schedule regular trims to remove split ends and promote healthy hair growth.
- **Hydration is Key**: Keep your hair moisturized by drinking plenty of water and using hydrating hair products.
- **Avoid Heat Styling**: Excessive heat styling can damage curly and coily hair. Limit the use of hot tools and opt for heatless styling methods.
- **Gentle Hair Care**: Use a gentle, sulfate-free shampoo and conditioner to avoid stripping your hair of its natural oils.

Sealing the Deal: Locking in Moisture with Castor Oil

One of the biggest challenges for those with curly and coily hair is maintaining moisture. Dry, brittle hair is more prone to breakage, split ends, and frizz. Castor oil, with its rich fatty acid content, is an excellent tool for sealing in moisture and preventing hair breakage.

Sealing the hair cuticle is essential for retaining moisture and preventing water loss. When the hair cuticle is open, moisture can easily escape, leaving the hair dry and brittle. By sealing the cuticle, you can lock in moisture, reduce frizz, and enhance shine.

The Role of Castor Oil in Sealing

Castor oil acts as a natural sealant, creating a protective barrier around the hair shaft. This barrier helps to prevent moisture loss and protect the hair from environmental damage. Here's how to use castor oil to seal in moisture:

1. **The L.C.O. Method**:

   - **Leave-in Conditioner**: Apply a generous amount of leave-in conditioner to damp hair, focusing on the ends.
   - **Curl Cream or Gel**: Apply your preferred styling product to define your curls and provide hold.
   - **Castor Oil Seal**: Finish by applying a small amount of castor oil to the ends of your hair. This will seal in moisture and prevent frizz.

2. **The L.C.O.M. Method**:

- **Leave-in Conditioner**: Apply a leave-in conditioner to damp hair.
- **Curl Cream or Gel**: Style your hair as desired.
- **Oil**: Apply a light oil, such as argan oil or jojoba oil, to the mid-lengths and ends of your hair.
- **Castor Oil Seal**: Finish by sealing the ends with a small amount of castor oil.

Tips for Effective Sealing

- **Warm the Oil**: Slightly warming the castor oil can enhance its penetration into the hair shaft.
- **Apply Sparingly**: A little castor oil goes a long way. Apply too much, and your hair may become greasy.
- **Focus on the Ends**: Concentrate on sealing the ends of your hair, as they are the most prone to dryness and damage.
- **Regular Deep Conditioning**: Deep condition your hair regularly to keep it moisturized and healthy.
- **Protective Styles**: Opt for protective hairstyles, such as braids or twists, to minimize manipulation and prevent breakage.
- **Gentle Hair Care**: Use a gentle, sulfate-free shampoo and conditioner to avoid stripping your hair of its natural oils.
- **Avoid Heat Styling**: Excessive heat styling can damage the hair cuticle and lead to dryness and breakage.

Additional Tips for Preventing Hair Breakage

- **Gentle Hair Handling:** Avoid rough handling, excessive brushing, and tight hairstyles.
- **Protective Styles:** Opt for protective hairstyles like braids, twists, or buns to minimize manipulation and breakage.
- **Regular Trims:** Schedule regular trims to remove split ends and prevent further damage.
- **Sleep on a Silk Pillowcase:** A silk pillowcase reduces friction, minimizing hair breakage.

By following these tips and incorporating castor oil into your hair care routine, you can effectively seal in moisture, reduce frizz, and achieve healthy, beautiful curls and coils.

Deep Conditioning with Castor Oil: A Luxurious Hair Treatment

Deep conditioning is a crucial step in any hair care routine, especially for curly and coily hair. It helps to restore moisture, strengthen the hair shaft, and improve overall hair health. Castor oil, with its rich fatty acid content, is an excellent ingredient for deep conditioning treatments.

The Benefits of a Castor Oil Hot Oil Treatment

- **Deep Hydration**: The heat from the warm oil helps to open the hair cuticle, allowing the castor oil to penetrate deeper into the hair shaft. This deep penetration provides intense hydration, leaving your hair soft, supple, and manageable.
- **Reduced Frizz**: By deeply conditioning the hair, castor oil helps to smooth the hair cuticle, reducing frizz and flyaways.
- **Strengthens Hair**: The nutrients in castor oil nourish the hair follicles, strengthening the hair shaft and preventing breakage.
- **Promotes Hair Growth**: Regular deep conditioning treatments with castor oil can stimulate blood circulation to the scalp, promoting hair growth.
- **Soothes the Scalp**: The warmth of the oil can help to soothe an irritated scalp, reducing itchiness and flakiness.

How to Perform a Castor Oil Hot Oil Treatment

1. **Warm the Oil**: Gently heat the castor oil, but avoid overheating it.
2. **Apply to Hair**: Section your hair and apply the warm oil to your scalp and hair, massaging gently.
3. **Cover and Wait**: Cover your hair with a shower cap or plastic wrap and let the oil sit for at least 30 minutes. For deeper conditioning, leave it on overnight.

4. **Shampoo and Condition**: Wash your hair with a gentle, sulfate-free shampoo to remove the oil. Follow up with a conditioner to restore moisture.

Additional Tips for a Luxurious Hot Oil Treatment

- **Combine Oils**: Mix castor oil with other hair-friendly oils like coconut oil, olive oil, or argan oil for added benefits.
- **Add Essential Oils**: Add a few drops of your favorite essential oil, such as lavender or rosemary, to enhance the aroma and therapeutic properties of the treatment.
- **Steam Your Hair**: For deeper penetration, cover your head with a hot towel or use a steamer while the oil is on your hair.
- **Regular Deep Conditioning**: Aim to do a deep conditioning treatment with castor oil once a week or every other week.
- **Protect Your Hair**: After a deep conditioning treatment, be gentle with your hair and avoid excessive heat styling.

Part IV

Total Well-being, Inside and Out

Chapter 6

A Healthier You: Castor Oil for Internal Cleansing and Detoxification

A Gentle Cleanse: Castor Oil for Digestive Health

Digestive health is a cornerstone of overall well-being. A healthy digestive system efficiently processes food, absorbs nutrients, and eliminates waste. When digestive issues arise, such as constipation, it can lead to discomfort and other health problems. Castor oil can be a valuable tool for promoting digestive health.

Castor oil's primary benefit for digestive health is its laxative effect. It works by stimulating the muscles in the intestines, promoting bowel movements and relieving constipation. The key component responsible for this effect is the ricinoleic acid.

How Castor Oil Works

- **Intestinal Stimulation**: Ricinoleic acid irritates the lining of the intestines, triggering a contraction of the intestinal muscles. This increased muscle activity helps to move stool through the digestive tract more efficiently.

- **Water Retention**: Castor oil can also increase water retention in the intestines, softening the stool and making it easier to pass.

Using Castor Oil for Digestive Health

When using castor oil as a laxative, it's crucial to follow the recommended dosage and consult with a healthcare professional, especially if you have any underlying health conditions. Here's a general guideline:

1. **Start with a Small Dose**: Begin with a small dose of castor oil, such as 1 teaspoon, and gradually increase it as needed.
2. **Mix with a Pleasant-Tasting Liquid**: To mask the unpleasant taste of castor oil, mix it with juice, water, or a smoothie.
3. **Monitor Your Body's Response**: Pay attention to your body's response to castor oil. It may take a few hours to work, so be patient.
4. **Drink Plenty of Water**: Drinking plenty of water helps to soften the stool and promote bowel movements.

Important Considerations:

- **Overuse**: Overusing castor oil can lead to dehydration and electrolyte imbalance.

- **Consult a Healthcare Professional**: If you experience persistent constipation or other digestive issues, consult a healthcare provider for proper diagnosis and treatment.
- **Pregnancy and Breastfeeding**: Pregnant and breastfeeding women should avoid using castor oil without consulting their healthcare provider.

Beyond Laxation:

While castor oil is primarily used for its laxative effects, it may offer additional benefits for digestive health:

- **Detoxification**: Some people believe that castor oil can help to cleanse the colon and remove toxins from the body.
- **Improved Nutrient Absorption**: By promoting regular bowel movements, castor oil can help to improve nutrient absorption.

By understanding the role of castor oil in supporting digestive health and using it appropriately, you can experience relief from constipation and improve your overall well-being.

A Natural Detox: Castor Oil for Liver Health

The liver, a vital organ, plays a crucial role in filtering toxins from the blood. Over time, exposure to environmental pollutants, poor diet, and stress can overburden the liver, leading to a buildup of toxins. Castor oil, with its unique properties, has been used for centuries to support liver health and promote detoxification.

Understanding the Liver's Role in Detoxification

The liver is responsible for processing and eliminating toxins from the body. It filters blood from the digestive tract, metabolizes drugs, and produces bile, which aids in digestion. When the liver becomes overwhelmed, it can lead to a variety of health problems, including fatigue, skin issues, and digestive disorders.

How Castor Oil Supports Liver Health

While more scientific research is needed to fully understand the mechanisms behind castor oil's liver-cleansing effects, traditional medicine and anecdotal evidence suggest several ways it may benefit the liver:

- Stimulates Bile Flow: Castor oil can stimulate the production and flow of bile, a substance produced by the liver that helps to break down fats and eliminate toxins.
- Improves Digestion: By promoting healthy digestion, castor oil can reduce the burden on the liver, allowing it to focus on detoxification.
- Antioxidant Properties: Some studies suggest that castor oil may have antioxidant properties, which can help to protect the liver from damage caused by oxidative stress.

Using Castor Oil for Liver Detoxification

To use castor oil for liver detoxification, you can incorporate it into your routine in the following ways:

- Castor Oil Packs: Apply a warm castor oil pack to your liver area, which is located on the right side of your abdomen, just below your ribs. This can help to stimulate liver function and promote detoxification.
- Internal Use: While not commonly recommended, some people use castor oil internally as a laxative. However, it's important to consult with a healthcare professional before trying this method.

Important Considerations

- Consult a Healthcare Professional: Before using castor oil for liver detoxification, it's essential to consult with a healthcare professional, especially if you have any underlying health conditions.
- Start Slowly: Begin with a small dose of castor oil and gradually increase it as needed.
- Monitor Your Body's Response: Pay attention to your body's reaction to castor oil. If you experience any adverse effects, discontinue use and consult a healthcare provider.
- Lifestyle Factors: In addition to using castor oil, focus on a healthy lifestyle, including a balanced diet, regular exercise, and adequate sleep.

By incorporating castor oil into your wellness routine and adopting healthy lifestyle habits, you can support your liver's natural detoxification processes and promote overall well-being.

A Slimmer You: Castor Oil and Weight Loss

While castor oil is primarily known for its laxative properties and skin benefits, some people believe it can also aid in weight loss and metabolism. While scientific research on this topic is limited, traditional medicine and anecdotal evidence suggest that castor oil may offer certain benefits.

How Castor Oil Might Aid Weight Loss

1. **Stimulates Digestion**: Castor oil's laxative properties can help to stimulate digestion and improve bowel function. A healthy digestive system is essential for efficient nutrient absorption and waste elimination.
2. **Detoxification**: By promoting regular bowel movements, castor oil can help to remove toxins from the body. This can lead to reduced bloating and a flatter stomach.
3. **Reduced Appetite**: Some people report feeling less hungry after using castor oil. This may be due to the

cleansing effect on the digestive system and the feeling of fullness it can provide.

Tips for Using Castor Oil for Weight Loss

If you're considering using castor oil for weight loss, it's essential to consult with a healthcare professional to discuss your specific needs and goals. Here are some general tips:

- **Internal Use**: Consume a small amount of castor oil mixed with a liquid, such as juice or water. However, it's crucial to follow the recommended dosage and consult with a healthcare provider before using castor oil internally.
- **External Use**: Apply castor oil topically to the abdomen to stimulate the digestive system and promote detoxification.
- **Healthy Diet and Exercise**: Combine the use of castor oil with a balanced diet and regular exercise for optimal weight loss results

Important Considerations

- **Consult a Healthcare Professional**: Before using castor oil for weight loss, consult with a healthcare provider to discuss your specific needs and goals.
- **Not a Magic Solution**: Castor oil is not a magic solution for weight loss. It should be used in conjunction with a healthy diet and regular exercise.

- **Potential Side Effects**: Overusing castor oil can lead to dehydration, electrolyte imbalance, and other side effects. It's important to use it in moderation and under the guidance of a healthcare professional.

Cautionary Note

While castor oil can be a helpful tool for supporting weight loss efforts, it's important to approach it with caution and consult with a healthcare professional. Excessive use of castor oil can lead to dehydration, electrolyte imbalance, and other health issues.

It's crucial to remember that sustainable weight loss is a journey that requires a holistic approach, including a balanced diet, regular exercise, and adequate sleep. Castor oil can be a complementary tool, but it should not be relied upon as a standalone solution.

Chapter 7

Pain Relief, Naturally: Castor Oil for Aches and Pains

Soothing Inflammation: The Anti-Inflammatory Power of Castor Oil

Pain and inflammation are common ailments that can significantly impact our quality of life. While there are many over-the-counter pain relievers available, many people are turning to natural alternatives, such as castor oil.

Castor oil's anti-inflammatory properties are primarily attributed to its main component, ricinoleic acid. This fatty acid has been shown to inhibit the production of inflammatory substances, such as prostaglandins and leukotrienes. By reducing inflammation, castor oil can help to alleviate pain and promote healing.

How Castor Oil Can Help Reduce Pain and Swelling

- **Muscle and Joint Pain**: Castor oil can be applied topically to alleviate pain associated with arthritis, muscle soreness, and joint inflammation. The anti-inflammatory properties of ricinoleic acid help to reduce swelling and discomfort.

- **Headaches and Migraines**: Applying a warm castor oil pack to the forehead or temples can help to relieve tension headaches and migraines. The warmth and soothing properties of castor oil can help to relax the muscles and reduce pain.
- **Back Pain**: A castor oil pack applied to the lower back can help to alleviate back pain caused by muscle tension or inflammation.
- **Menstrual Cramps**: Castor oil can help to reduce menstrual cramps by relaxing the uterine muscles.

Using Castor Oil for Pain Relief

There are several ways to use castor oil for pain relief:

- **Topical Application**: Apply a warm castor oil pack directly to the affected area. Cover the pack with a heating pad or warm cloth to enhance its therapeutic effects.
- **Massage**: Gently massage castor oil into the affected area to improve blood circulation and reduce pain and inflammation.
- **Bath Additives**: Add a few drops of castor oil to your bathwater to soothe sore muscles and joints.

Important Considerations

While castor oil is generally safe for topical use, it's important to use it correctly and consult with a healthcare professional if you have any underlying health conditions.

- **Patch Test**: Before applying castor oil to a large area of skin, perform a patch test to check for any allergic reactions.
- **Avoid Open Wounds**: Do not apply castor oil to open wounds or broken skin.
- **Pregnancy and Breastfeeding**: Pregnant and breastfeeding women should consult with a healthcare provider before using castor oil.

The Healing Power of Castor Oil Packs

Castor oil packs are a traditional remedy that has been used for centuries to relieve pain and inflammation. By applying a warm castor oil pack to the pain affected area, you can soothe sore muscles, reduce joint pain, and promote healing.

Understanding the Benefits of Castor Oil Packs

- **Increased Blood Flow**: The heat from the castor oil pack helps to increase blood flow to the affected area, delivering oxygen and nutrients to the tissues.

- **Reduced Inflammation**: Castor oil has anti-inflammatory properties that can help to reduce swelling and pain.
- **Pain Relief**: By reducing inflammation and increasing blood flow, castor oil packs can help to alleviate pain.
- **Improved Lymphatic Drainage**: Castor oil packs can stimulate the lymphatic system, helping to remove toxins and waste products from the body.

How to Perform a Castor Oil Pack

Materials Needed:

- Castor oil
- Flannel cloth or cotton cloth
- Plastic wrap
- Heating pad or hot water bottle

Instructions:

1. **Warm the Oil**: Gently heat the castor oil. Avoid overheating, as excessive heat can damage the skin.
2. **Soak the Cloth**: Dip the flannel cloth or cotton cloth into the warm castor oil. Make sure the cloth is well-saturated.
3. **Apply the Pack**: Place the oil-soaked cloth on the affected area. For example, if you have lower back pain, place the cloth on your lower back.

4. **Cover the Pack**: Cover the cloth with plastic wrap to prevent the oil from staining your clothes or bedding.
5. **Apply Heat**: Place a heating pad or hot water bottle over the plastic wrap to maintain heat.
6. **Leave it On**: Leave the castor oil pack on for at least 30 minutes. For optimal results, you can leave it on for up to an hour.
7. **Remove the Pack**: Gently remove the pack and clean the area with a damp cloth.

Tips for Effective Castor Oil Packs

- **Skin Sensitivity**: If you have sensitive skin, test the castor oil on a small area of skin before applying it to a larger area.
- **Personalize Your Treatment**: You can customize your castor oil pack by adding essential oils, such as lavender or peppermint, to enhance the therapeutic benefits.
- **Hydrate**: Drink plenty of water to stay hydrated, especially after using a castor oil pack.
- **Consult a Healthcare Professional**: If you have a chronic condition or severe pain, consult with a healthcare professional before using castor oil packs.

Part V

Your Journey to Holistic Health

When to Avoid Castor Oil

- **Pregnancy**: Pregnant women should avoid using castor oil, especially in the later stages of pregnancy, as it can stimulate uterine contractions.
- **Breastfeeding**: While there is limited information on the effects of castor oil during breastfeeding, it's best to consult with a healthcare provider before using it.
- **Infants and Children**: Castor oil should not be used in infants and young children without medical supervision.
- **People with Certain Medical Conditions**: Individuals with inflammatory bowel disease, irritable bowel syndrome, or other digestive disorders should consult with a healthcare provider before using castor oil.

Debunking Myths: The Truth About Castor Oil

Castor oil has been used for centuries as a natural remedy for various ailments. However, there are several myths and misconceptions surrounding its safety and efficacy. Let's debunk some of these common myths and explore the facts.

Myth 1: Castor Oil is Toxic

One of the most persistent myths about castor oil is that it is toxic. This misconception likely stems from the fact that castor beans, the source of castor oil, contain a toxic substance called ricin. However, the process of extracting castor oil removes ricin, making the final product safe for use.

Myth 2: Castor Oil Can Cause Infertility

There is no scientific evidence to support the claim that castor oil can cause infertility. In fact, some traditional medicine practices have used castor oil to promote fertility. However, it's important to use castor oil responsibly and consult with a healthcare provider if you have any concerns.

Myth 3: Castor Oil is Only for Laxative Purposes

While castor oil is often associated with its laxative effects, it has a wide range of other uses. It can be used topically for skin and hair care, as well as internally for digestive health and detoxification.

Myth 4: Castor Oil Can Cause Addiction

There is no evidence to suggest that castor oil is addictive. It is a natural substance that can be used safely and effectively when used as directed.

Fact-Checking Castor Oil

To dispel these myths, it's essential to rely on scientific evidence and reputable sources of information. Here are some key facts about castor oil:

- **Safe for Topical Use**: Castor oil is generally safe for topical use on the skin and hair.
- **Internal Use Requires Caution**: When used internally, castor oil can have strong laxative effects. It's important to use it in moderation and under the guidance of a healthcare provider.
- **Consult a Healthcare Professional**: Before using castor oil, especially internally, consult with a healthcare provider to ensure it's safe and appropriate for your individual needs.

www.ingramcontent.com/pod-product-compliance
Lightning Source LLC
Chambersburg PA
CBHW061306250726
48653CB00002B/798